Stress Management for Beginners

Simple Techniques, Methods, and Skills for a Healthier Stress Free Life

By Martin Redman

If you find this book helpful, please leave a review on Amazon [here][1] . It will help others also find this book.

---

[1] http://www.powerlists.org/qq1q

Table of Contents

A Free E-Book for You

As a token of my appreciation for your purchasing this book, I want to offer you a free e-book:

"You've Got (Too Much) Mail! 38 Do's and Don'ts To Tame Your Inbox"

This e-book is the third book in the bestselling PowerLists™ book series and offers 38 of the best practices for handling e-mails.

>>>Tap Here to Grab Your Free E-Book <<<[2]

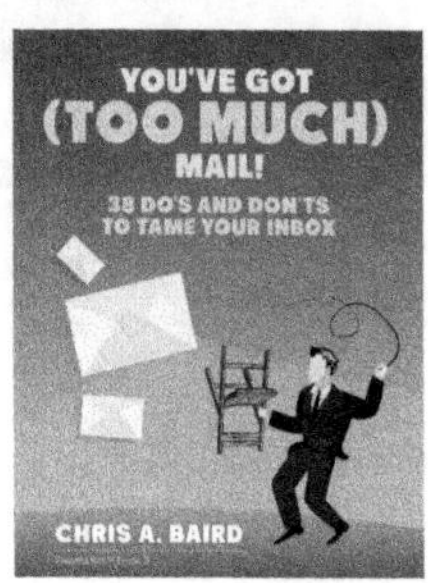

---

[2] http://www.powerlists.org/s9si

1 - Introduction

Stress

Stress is a part of almost everyone's life in one form or the other. While at first glance, it might seem like a bad thing or phenomenon, it is not entirely bad. Stress helps to keep us on our toes as well as serve as a drive in the pursuit of our goals.

However, too much of it is not good for the body as it starts to affect us negatively. This is because when an individual is stressed, focusing on work becomes difficult. It starts affecting your relationship with the people in your life like your spouse, children, friends or other family members.

You also tend to pick up bad habits easily once you are stressed. This is because you feel they are an outlet for releasing the stress. This is not really true but is just a trick your mind is playing on you. Some of these bad habits include:

- Smoking

- Excessive drinking

- Regular arguments and fights with those around you

- Overeating which will lead to weight gain

- Regularly getting lost in thought

- Using pills or drugs to relax

- Sleeping too much

- Taking out your stress on others

All these habits never bring out the best in people due to the stress they are going through. In fact, a lot of times, people just tend to be stressed over unnecessary things or over the smallest of problems. This may happen when they can't just calm down and clear their mind to find a possible solution to whatever is causing the stress.

Like I said earlier, stress is a part of our lives and I am not so sure that stress can or should be entirely eliminated due to the good purpose it serves. However, just like our emotions, stress needs to be kept in check and this book will be examining how to do just that. So come along with me and let us show you how to control stress rather than the other way round.

2 - What is Stress Management?

Definition

Stress management can be defined as the techniques, methods or skills used to deal with or reduce stress. Considering the fact that stress cannot be completely eliminated, it can be reduced to a minimum such that it will not interfere with:

- Our daily activities

- Family time

- Work

- Relationships

- Our own leisure time for relaxation

Stress management starts with recognizing the source of stress in your life. Then, steps can then be taken to control it just like a doctor diagnoses the illness of a patient before prescribing drugs for him or her.

3 - Methods for Coping

There is no one particular solution to stress management since we all have different reactions to stress. However, there are still some basic steps that can be taken by an individual experiencing stress. After recognizing the source of stress in your life, you can do the following:

Take adequate care of yourself

Change the stressful situation which could be possible if it is your job or the area you are living in.

Change your reaction

This is especially effective when it is family or a dating relationship which will reduce the possibility of arguments and reduce the potential for stress.

Set Aside Time for Rest

Start setting aside time for rest and relaxation as this will keep your mind and head clear such that you will not end up making the wrong decisions. Even when the stress comes around again, your reaction is different which will go a long way in reducing the potential for increase in the level of the stress.

If you are really suffering from stress and you want to reduce it, you need to learn how to write things down. This may involve keeping a diary to write things down about the stress-causing situations or events. This will allow you to adequately manage the stress.

Major life-changing events can trigger high stress such as:

- Changing of jobs

- Relocating to a new place to live

- Losing a loved one

- Suffering a serious accident

It is easy to identify those as likely causes of stress but then how about those events that cause you stress on a regular basis without the involvement of a major negative event. Well, this is where the diary comes in handy. You use it to track your causes of stress and the patterns that it takes.

In the diary, you ask yourself the following questions and then try and provide an answer to them:

- Do you explain stress as temporary? Something like "I just have a lot I am dealing with right now" even though it's been a while that you have taken time to relax

- Do you view stress as an integral part of your work or home with statements like "every day here is hectic" or maybe as part of your personality like "I just seem to have a lot of energy, that's all"

- What is the cause of your stress?

- How did you feel both physically and emotionally?

- What was your response to the stress?

- What did you do to get over it when it happened?

Answering these questions will help you to gain an understanding of how to begin to cope with the stress in your life. Most likely it will reduce it so that it does not get out of control which could really spell trouble for such an individual.

You need to start accepting responsibility for the role you yourself play as an individual in the creation or maintenance of stress. That is because a lot of us tend to get worked up over the minutest of things. It is imperative that we keep our stress under check.

This will allow us to enjoy living life as well as enjoying our relationships with those around us. We will still examine some steps in details but we should never allow stress to overcome or take over our lives.

4 - How Does Stress Work?

As earlier stated, stress can be a useful element but only to certain point. After that it becomes harmful and no more serves a beneficial purpose. Basically, stress is the reaction or response of the body to any form of threat or demand.

Physical Response

Whenever there is a form of threat, the nervous system responds by releasing stress hormones like adrenaline and cortisol which then stimulates the body for action. This, then, causes:

- A rise in blood pressure

- Tightening of muscles

- Quickening of breath

- An increase in the sharpness of senses

These, together, bring about an increase in strength and stamina, increased speed of reaction time and enhancement of focus. If it is needed, it drives and motivates you towards success. This is because your brain becomes sharp and you know that you need to get that thing done due to the success or glory it will bring you.

Stress drives students to excel on their exams and be better than their peers. Stress drives politicians to do everything within their power to win elections and stand out among other candidates vying for a particular office. It is also stress that drives people towards excellence in their places of work such that they are exceptional and unique among other workers in that same workplace.

Stress something of a motivator or catalyst since it tends to drive people toward something. That is towards a change from the present situation. However, when it starts crossing a particular threshold it starts producing the wrong results or bad habits in a person. Then it needs to be checked.

Sometimes even the excitement of a new change can bring stress. This may include the feeling people experience whenever they are about to get married which is commonly referred to as wedding jitters. So just like life, stress has a good and a bad side and definitely needs to be kept in check or controlled.

5 - Research

From research, it has been pointed out that there are three major ways by which we respond to stress and they are:

Social engagement

This seems to be the relatively easiest way of responding to stress as it allows us to be calm and feel safe with little or no effort. This involves interacting with people. It may be just talking to them about a particular problem that you are facing in order to help keep you calm and collected.

This then allows you to have a clear mind to shape out an eventual solution to the problem. This helps to eliminate the stress. Guess they were right when they said, "problem shared is half-solved".

Mobilization

This is also known as the fight or flight response. This usually comes up when there is danger or we feel threatened by something. It doesn't even matter whether the threat is real or just registered in our subconscious (superficial). Either way the body consequently responds by releasing hormones that fit the situation noticeably adrenaline.

In such situations, systems like the digestive and immune system stop functioning temporarily at this point with the immune system switching into action until you are either able to fight or run. When the stress finally passes, the nervous system calms the body down and normal functions return.

Immobilization

This is the least applied of responses and the least enjoyable as it is employed only when the first two have failed. Usually for extreme life-threatening situations in which you find yourself in a traumatized or dysfunctional state unable to move this kicks in.

Sometimes, you might even lose consciousness such that you are able to withstand high levels of physical pain. While it is easy for the nervous system to return the body to its normal function in the first two responses.

It is a little difficult in this response as the body is going to need stimulation by the individual. This means that there needs to be a realization of the state that such an individual is before he or she can come out of such state.

6 - The Four Consequences of Ignoring Stress

They say "what you do not know does not kill you" but this isn't true. When you see or observe stress in your life but then decide to do nothing about it and prefer to ignore it, you are taking an unnecessary risk. This may even put your life in a precarious situation.

When you ignore stress such that it keeps occurring over and over again, then you are exposing yourself to death-causing situations. This is because the hormone cortisol which is released when we are stressed begins to accumulate in the bloodstream which causes the major problem.

Decreased immune function

When stress accumulates as a result of ignoring it, it affects the immune system as it is not able to protect us against illnesses which it normally shields us against. As such, we become susceptible to various bacterial and viral infections which could lead to more severe diseases.

Memory Problems

Too much of the hormone cortisol due to accumulation of stress has a damaging effect on the brain. It brings about deterioration of the hippocampus in the brain that can lead to memory loss which could signify Alzheimer's disease.

Heart attack

With high level of stress, there is constant rising of the blood pressure which means increased and more than necessary amount of blood is pumped to the heart which consequently increases the possibility of heart attack.

Obesity

Prolonged stress and the effect of the actions of cortisol on the body can lead to obesity. This has been linked to heart disease as a result of high blood pressure and cholesterol. Furthermore, people suffering from obesity have been shown to be at the risk of type II diabetes and various types of cancer. So, watch out for that stress and keep it in check.

7 - Tricks for Managing Stress

Our reactions to situations all differ and vary from one individual to the next. There are various ways by which stress can be managed and while all methods might not elicit the same reaction in everybody, you need to find the one that works best for you.

Then you need to apply it in order to manage and reduce the stress in your life. Here are some ways of managing stress.

Adopt a healthy lifestyle

The way you live will determine how well you will cope with stress. Basically, your diet is important as well as whatever you decide to put in your tummy.

Diet

You can start by eating a healthy diet since well-nourished bodies are able to cope better with stress compared to poorly nourished bodies. So ensure your diet is a balanced one.

Caffeine and sugar

Another thing to do is to reduce the amount of caffeine and sugar that you consume as the initial excitement they produce ends in a low level energy and bad mood. Furthermore, this will lead to getting better amount of sleep which means no room for stress.

Alcohol, cigarettes and drugs

Avoid alcohol, cigarettes and drugs as they do you little or no good. Fine, they may relieve you of stress in the short-term but in the long-term. The stress will come back stronger. Also they tend to cloud the mind of an individual.

Sleep

Ensure you get enough sleep as sleep allows the brain to rest. It also clears the mind of clogs and obstacles such that when you wake up, you feel relaxed and balanced. This then allows you to tackle the problems objectively and smartly.

Engage in physical activity

Physical activity is activity that involves movement and

raises your heart rate. Exercising is great for your health and it releases endorphins which are good hormones that help keep the stress out. One good thing about exercise is that almost anyone can engage in it and you do not need to be an athlete.

While exercising, do not focus on the stressors in your life. Rather, focus on the sensation you are feeling while carrying out the exercise. Also, choose an activity that suits you most. This will allow you to enjoy it and to practice regularly which means lower levels of stress.

Social Engagement

This is the fastest, quickest and most efficient way of reducing stress. It also helps in being able to stop yourself from overreacting to seemingly problematic situations. This is because you get to communicate with another human being who understands and resonates with your situation. This has a calming effect like no other.

Ways of getting involved in social engagement include:

- Reaching out to a colleague at work

- Asking a loved one to check in on you regularly

- Helping people by volunteering

- Meeting new people by taking a class or joining a club

- Going for a walk with a companion

Avoid Unnecessary Stress

There are some forms of stress that you know are there and you are already familiar with. These kinds of stress should not give you problems. Rather, just avoid them or learn to accept them as the case may be.

If there is someone at your workplace that is always getting under your skin, just avoid them. If he or she is persistent, once the person starts, get ear muffs or listen to music through your headphones. Set a limit to what you will do and what you will not do. Never let people push you into something you don't want to do. Otherwise, will likely bring you stress.

Make Time for Fun and Relaxation

This is another important way you can reduce stress as your mind will be clear and taken off those stressors. You will get to smile and laugh. Laughter is considered to be good for the soul since you are stressed less, and you get to focus on the positives of life. So you should set aside time to relax, play, have fun and get together with family and friends. Basically just give yourself a break!

8 - What Does Life Without Stress Look Like?

A life with little or no stress is a wonderful and peaceful life. Such an individual is calm, collected and has a clear head when it comes to making decisions. He or she has no worries while focusing more on the good side of life rather than the bad because when you are stressed, all you will see is the negative side which will only compound the problem.

The Stress-Free Individual

A stress-free individual is objective in making decisions because he or she has no clogs when it comes to finding solutions to a problem. For such individuals, they do not run away when faced with problems. They usually see them as challenges that need to be overcome. So, instead of sulking and worrying themselves out, they smile, take a deep breath and look for solutions to the problems.

9 - Conclusion

Stress cannot be totally eliminated from life. However, it can be reduced to the barest minimum depending on how well you manage it. While there are various techniques for managing stress, you, as an individual, need to find the best one that resonates with you. Then, you can reduce the stress in your life.

Various forms of stressors exist depending on the situation an individual is facing. This is why you first need to understand yourself and the way you react to things. This will guide you on the best technique to apply in order to cure the stress.

Just clear your mind and take in nature, appreciate the beauty surrounding you. Take a deep breath and look forward to new things that are coming your way rather than the problem you are facing.

Value the people around you and try to share with them so that they can understand you and render the help they can to you so that you do not go through everything all alone. Stress can be reduced if you take charge and are ready to stop it from taking charge of or having control over you.

Thank You

As we reach the end of this book, I want to say thanks for reading this book.

I want to get this information out to as many people as possible. If you found this book helpful, I would greatly appreciate you leaving me a review on Amazon here[3] . This helps others find the book as well.

I love hearing from readers so please get in touch via E-mail: cabpublishing1@gmail.com[4]

------

[3]http://www.powerlists.org/qq1q

[4]mailto:cabpublishing1@gmail.com

Disclaimer

This document is geared towards providing exact and reliable information in regards to the topic and issue covered. The publication is sold with the idea that the publisher is not required to render accounting, officially permitted, or otherwise, qualified services. If advice is necessary, legal or professional, a practiced individual in the profession should be ordered.

This information is not presented by a medical practicioner and is for educational and informational purposes only. The content is not intended as a substitute for professional medical advice, diagnosis, or treatment. Always seek the advice of your physician or other qualified health care provider with any questions you may have regarding a medical condition. Never disregard professional medical advice or delay in seeking it because of something you have read.

The information provided herein is stated to be truthful and consistent, in that any liability, in terms of inattention or otherwise, by any usage or abuse of any policies, processes, or directions contained within is the solitary and utter responsibility of the recipient reader. Under no circumstances will any legal responsibility or blame be held against the

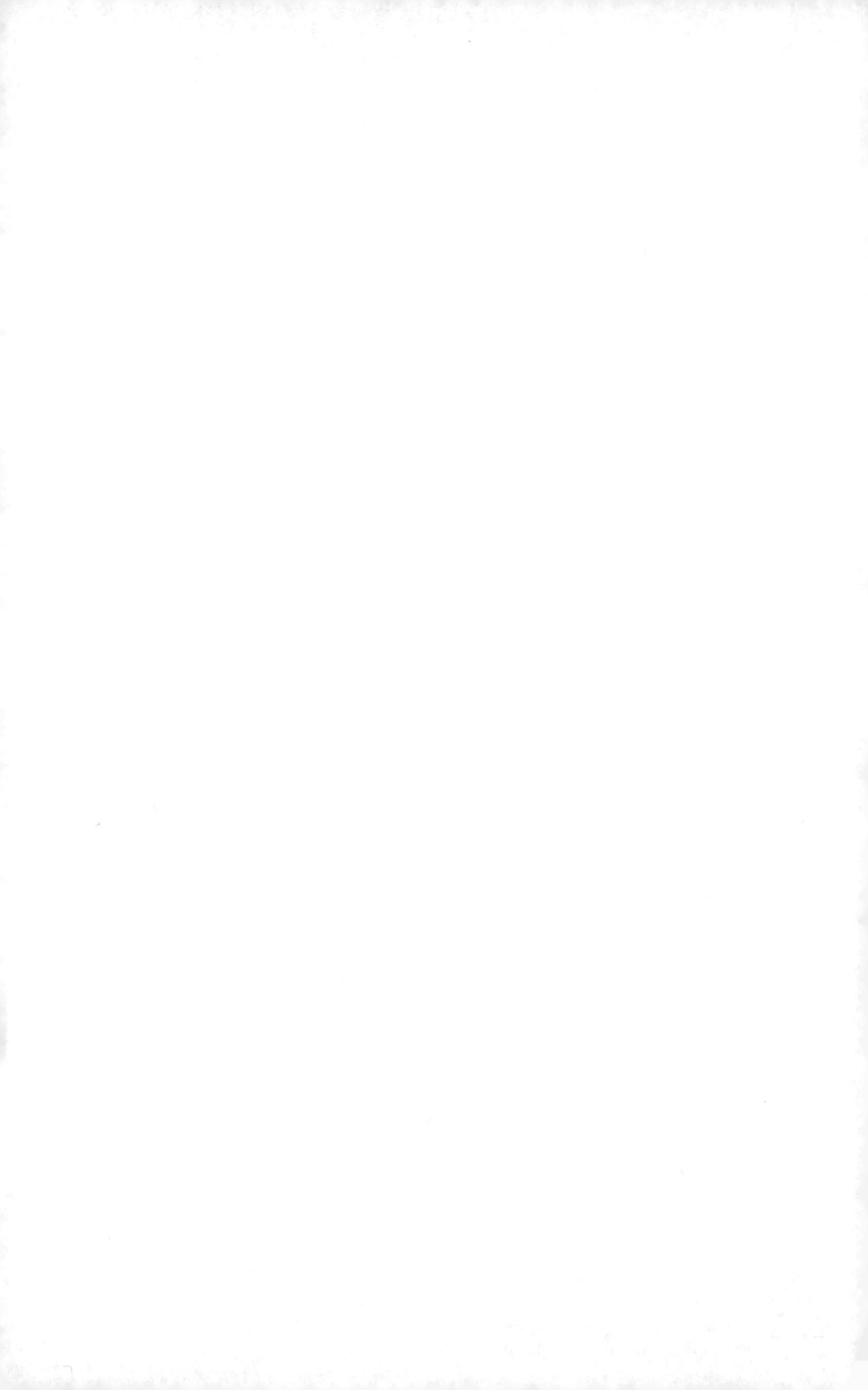